SAFETY FIRST!

OUTDOORS

By Eugene Baker
Pictures by Tom Dunnington

Zachary's WorkshopLTD • Creative Education

Published by Creative Education, Inc.,
123 South Broad Street, Mankato, Minnesota 56001
Copyright ©1980 by Creative Education, Inc.
International copyrights reserved in all countries.
No part of this book may be reproduced in any form without
written permission from the publisher.
Printed in the United States.

Created by "Zachary's Workshop Ltd."
Lake Forest, Illinois 60045

Library of Congress Cataloging in Publication Data
Baker, Eugene H.
    Safety first ... outdoors.
    SUMMARY: Presents safety tips for playing out of
doors.
    1. Play—Safety measures—Juvenile literature.
2. Recreation—Safety measures—Juvenile literature.
3. Amusements—Safety measures—Juvenile literature.
[1.Play—Safety measures. 2. Safety] I. Dunnington,
Tom. II. Title.
GV182.9.B34   614.8'77   79-25053   ISBN 0-87191-736-X lib. bdg.

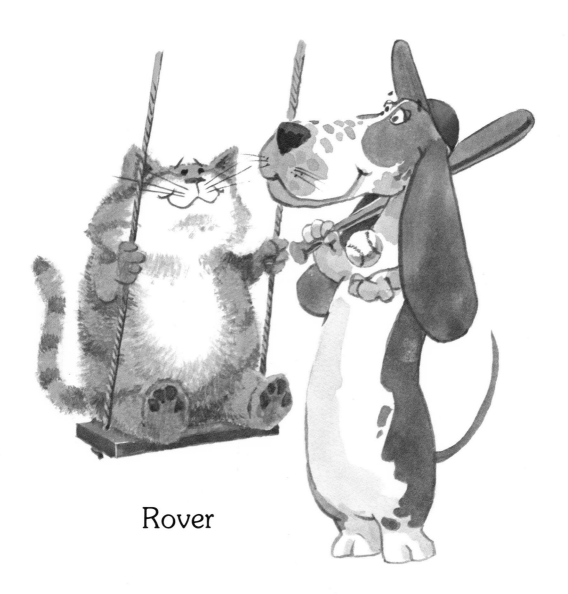

Rover

Basil

"Man on base," yelled Rover. "Get a hit, Basil!"

"I'll hit it past the street light," answered Basil.

Can you see what's wrong?

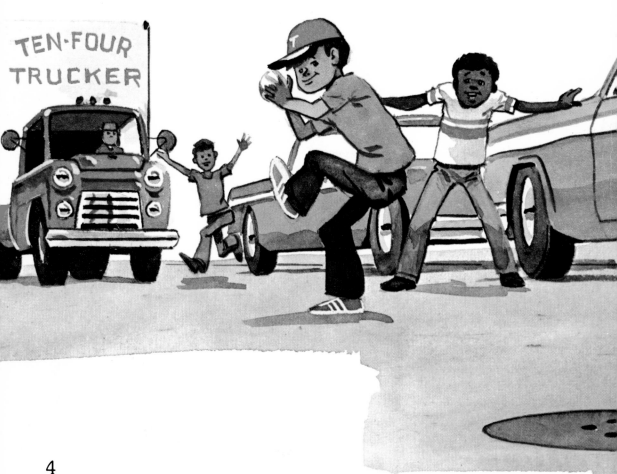

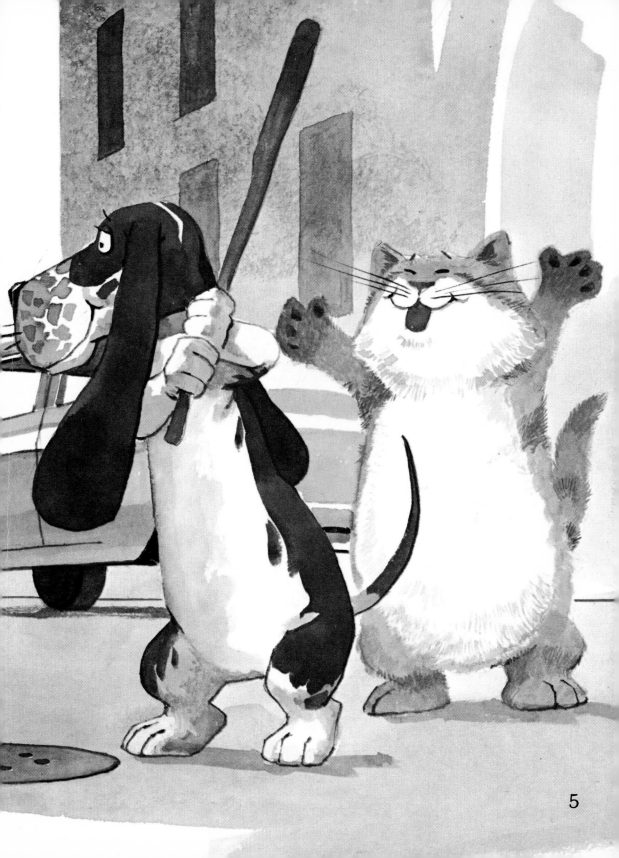

- Do not play in streets.
- Do not run out from between parked cars.
- Cross streets only at corners.
- Stop, look and listen before crossing.

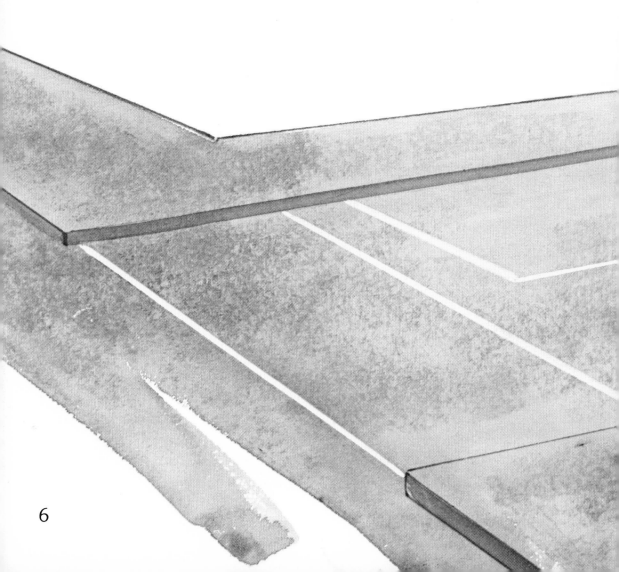

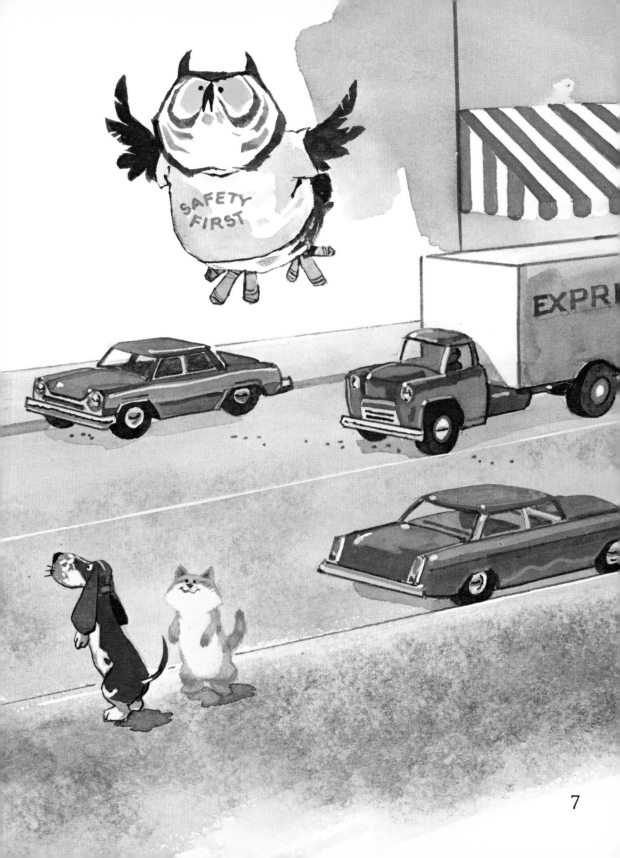

"I dare you to climb to the top of the swings," said Rover.

"That's easy!" said Basil.

Can you see what's wrong?

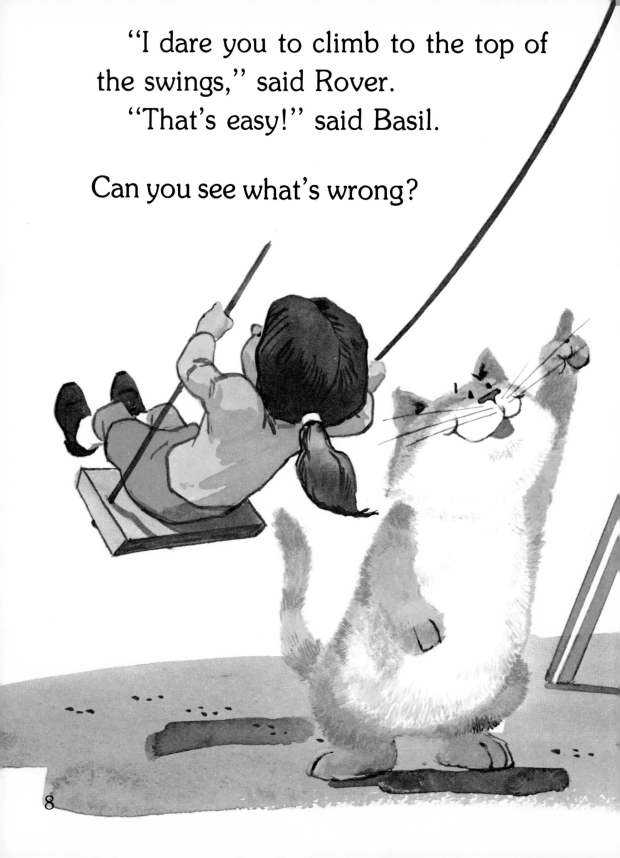

8

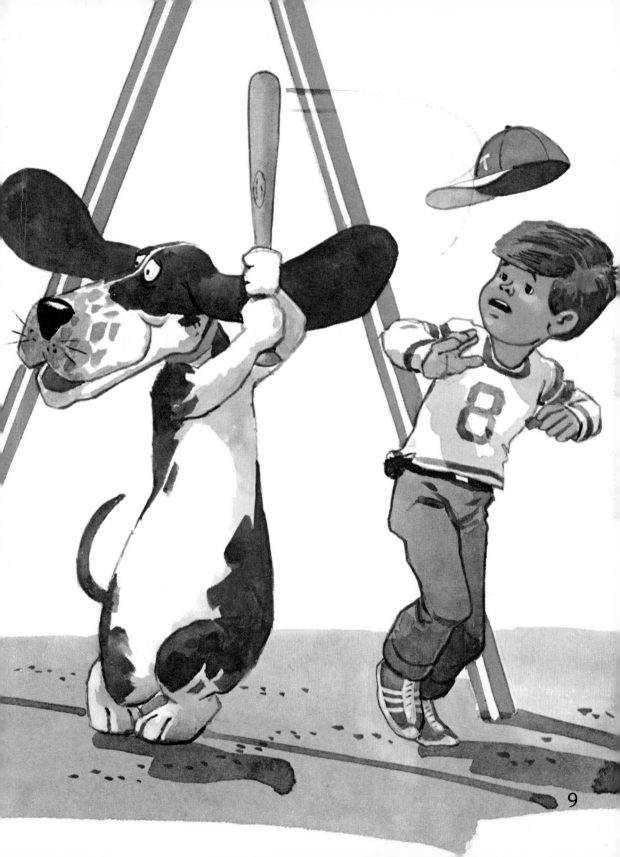

9

- Do not take dares to use play equipment in incorrect ways.
- Do not play behind or near swings.
- Watch for people around you when you swing a bat.
- Be careful when equipment is wet and slippery.

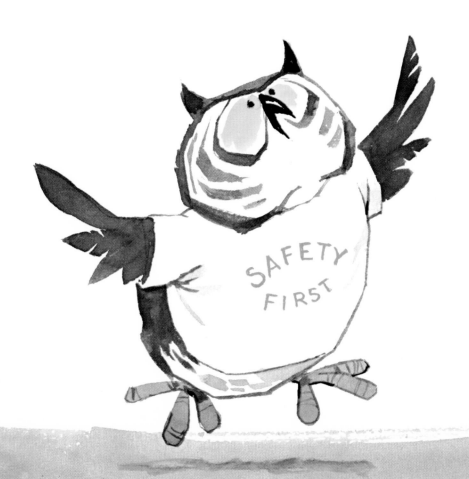

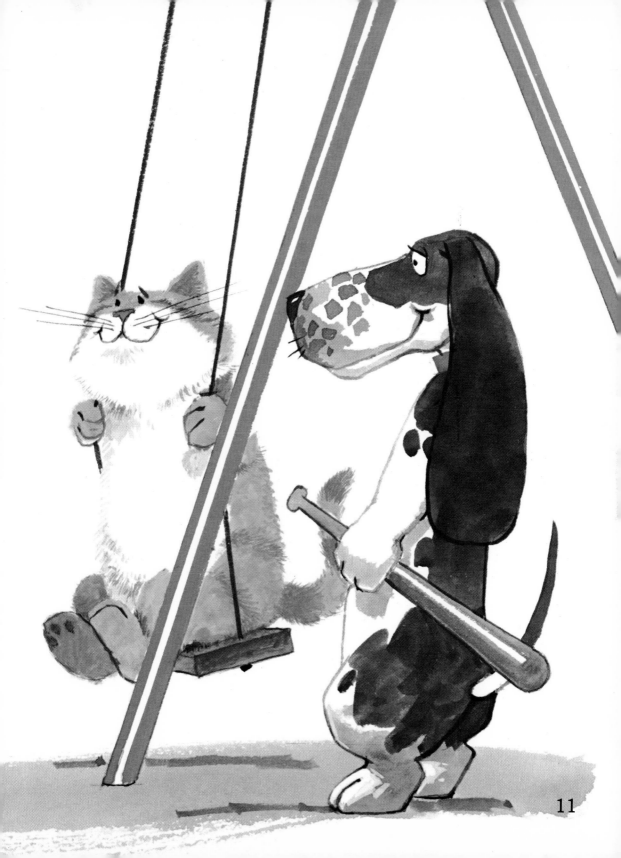

11

"This fence is higher than it looks," said Rover.

"Watch out for the sharp points on top," answered Basil.

Can you see what's wrong?

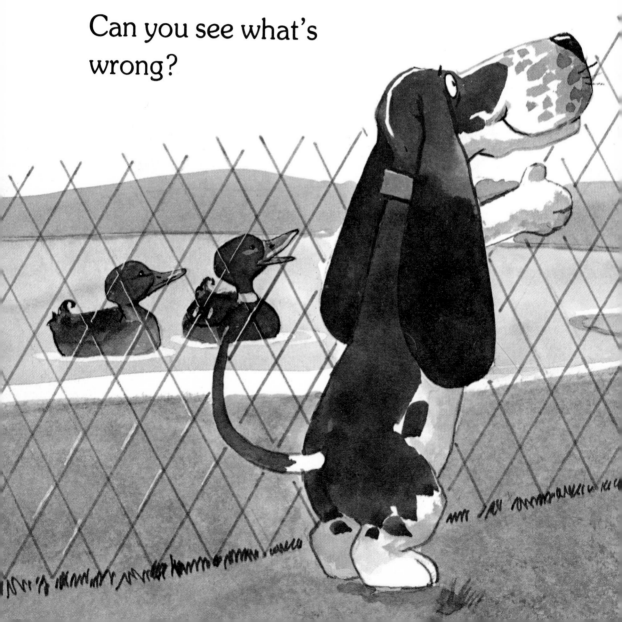

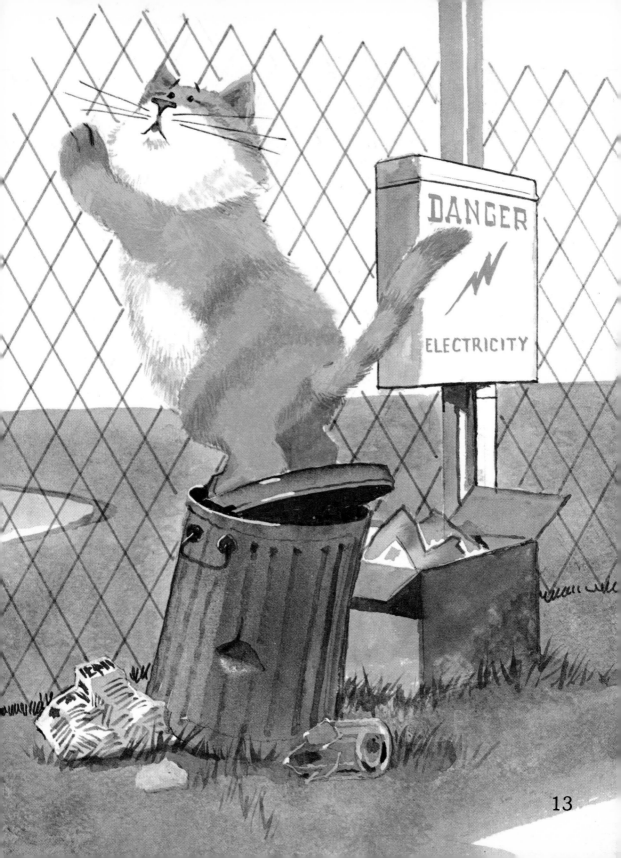

- Do not climb high fences.
- Stay away from trash cans and broken bottles.
- Stay away from electrical equipment.

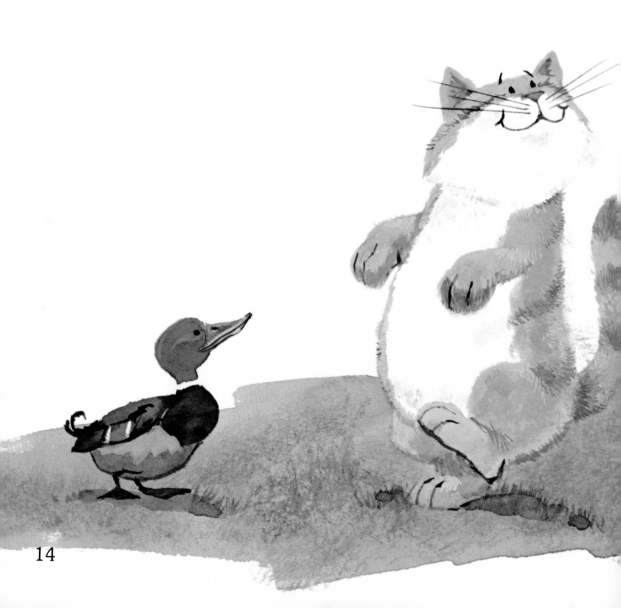

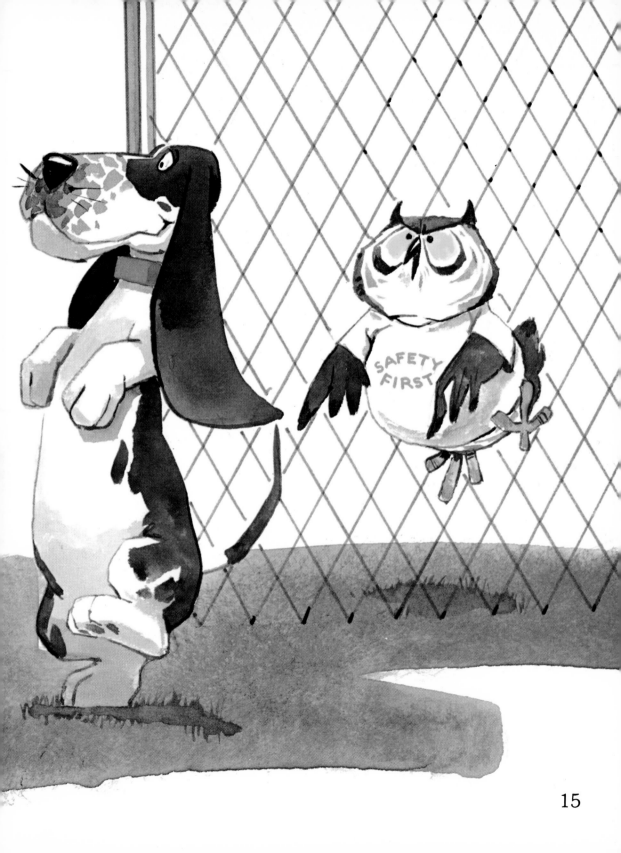

"What's inside that old big box?" asked Rover.

"It sure would be a great place to hide," answered Basil.

Can you see what's wrong?

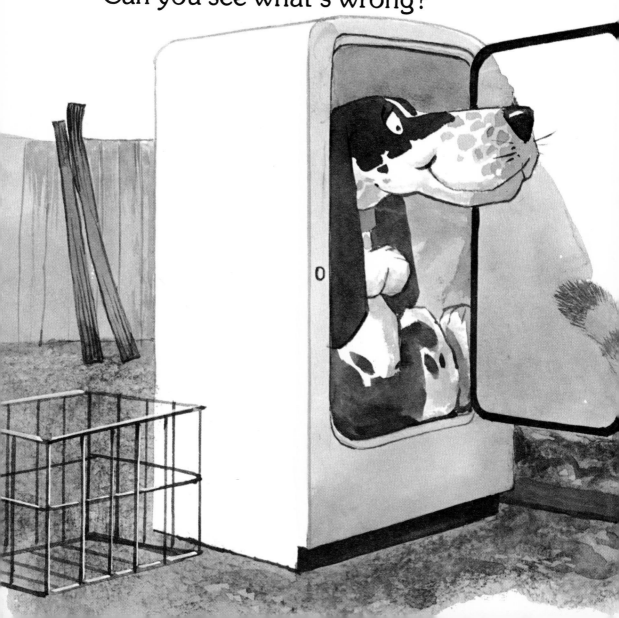

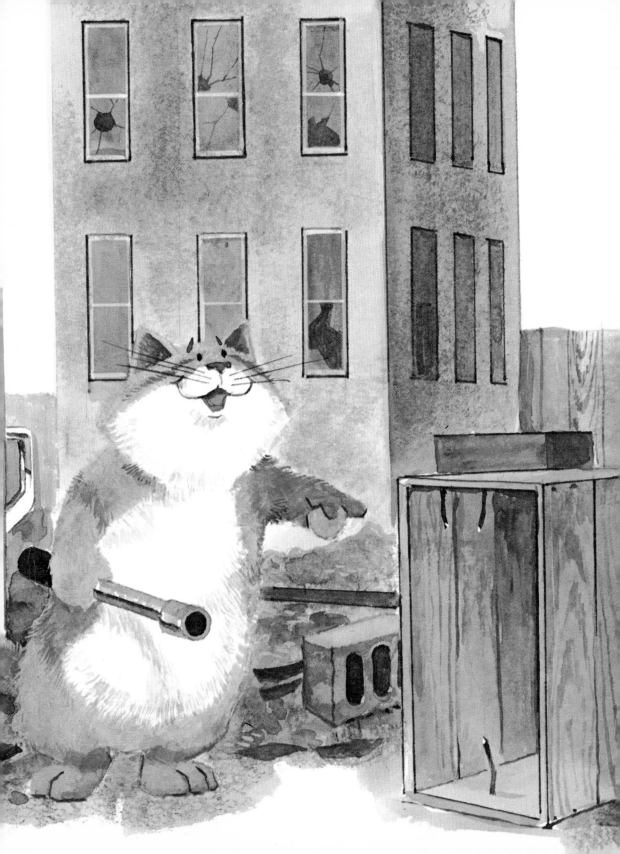

- Do not play in abandoned buildings.
- Do not play or hide in old trunks or refrigerators where lid or door can swing shut, trapping you inside.

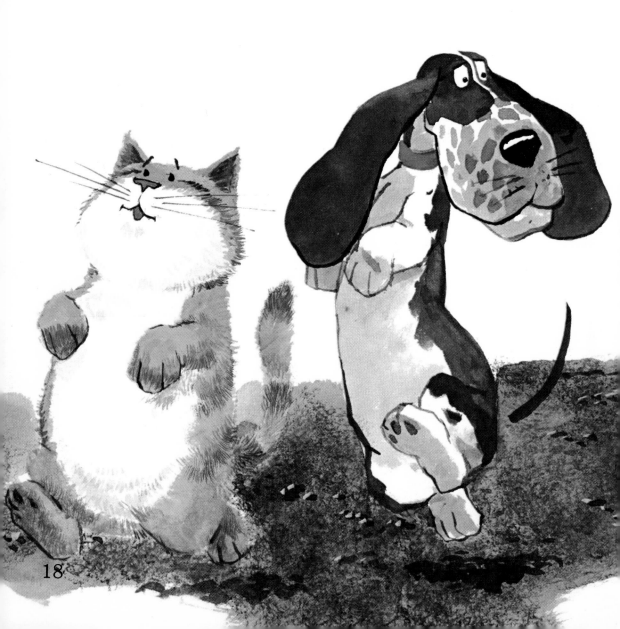

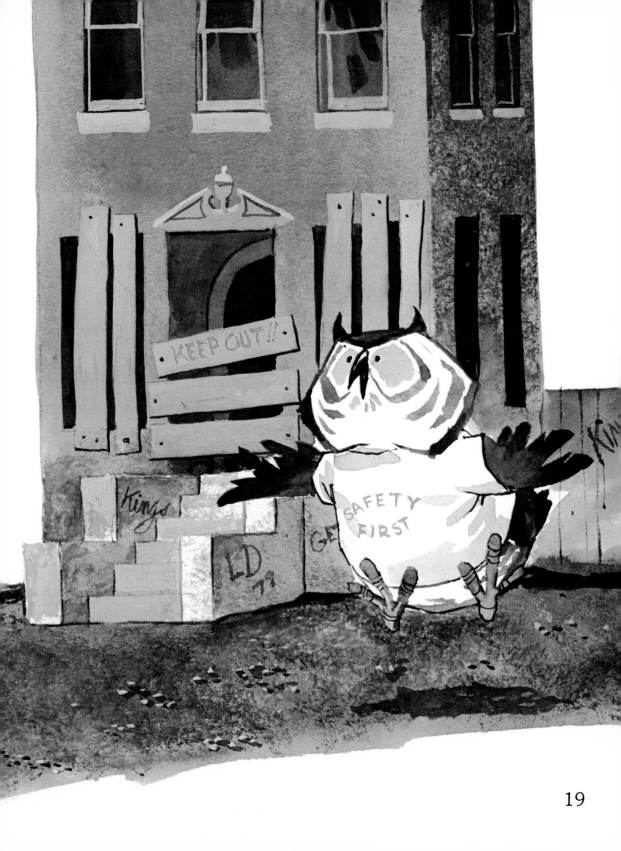

19

"Look out for the bait can,"
yelled Basil.

"Maybe the fishing is better near
shore," answered Rover.

Can you see what's wrong?

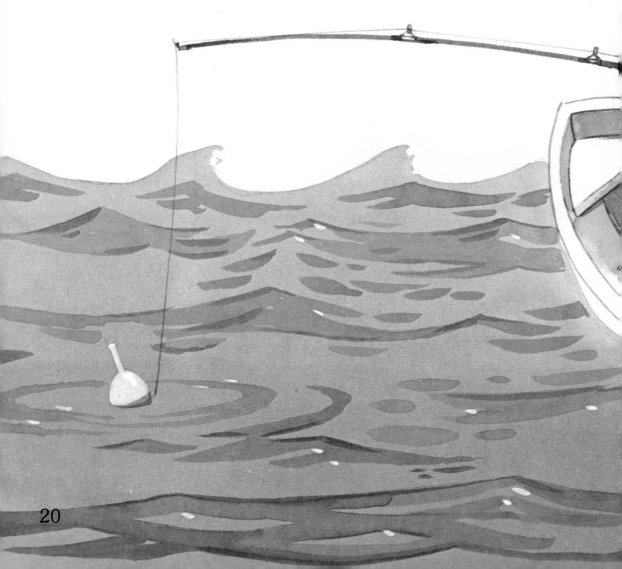

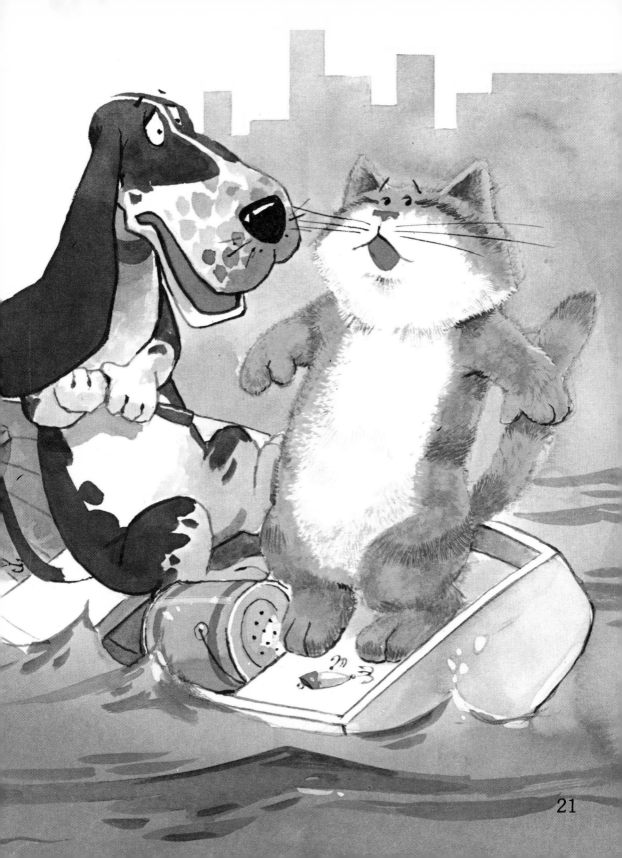

- Do not stand up in a boat.
- Be careful with fish hooks and knives.
- Come back to shore when the water gets rough.
- Look where you step when fishing on a pier.

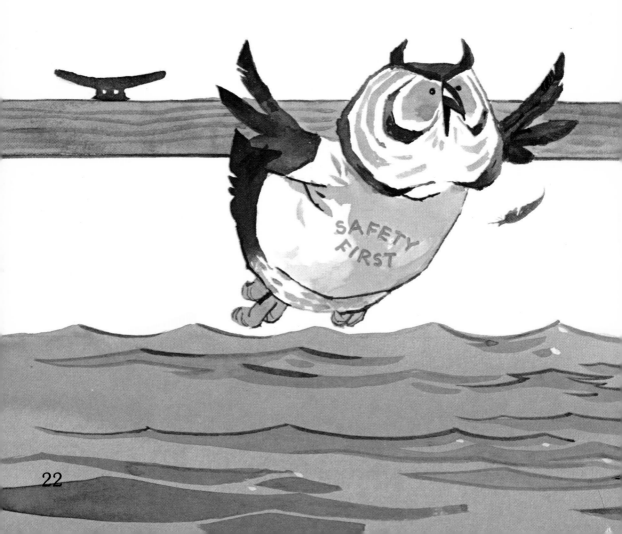

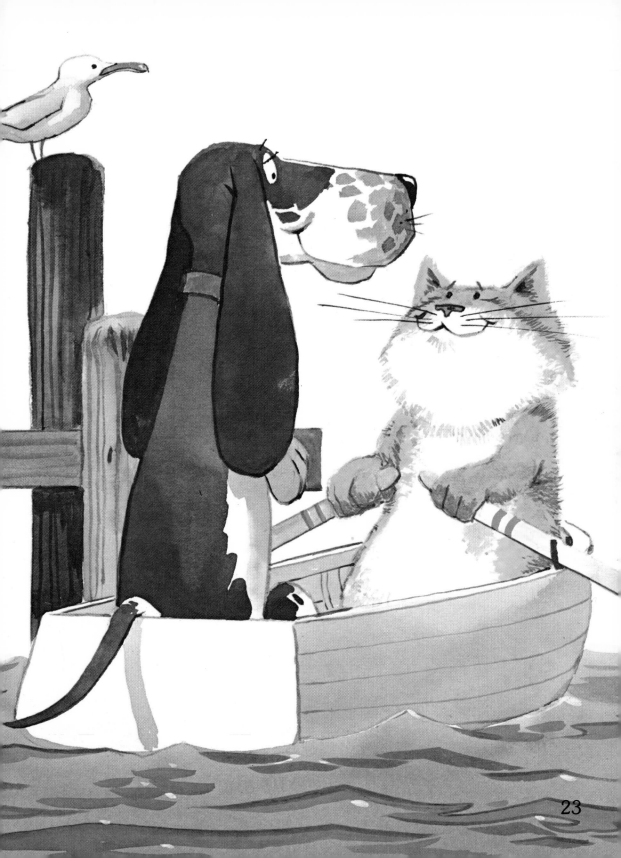

23

"How do you like your new teacher?" asked Basil.

"Not as much as recess," smiled Rover.

Can you see what's wrong?

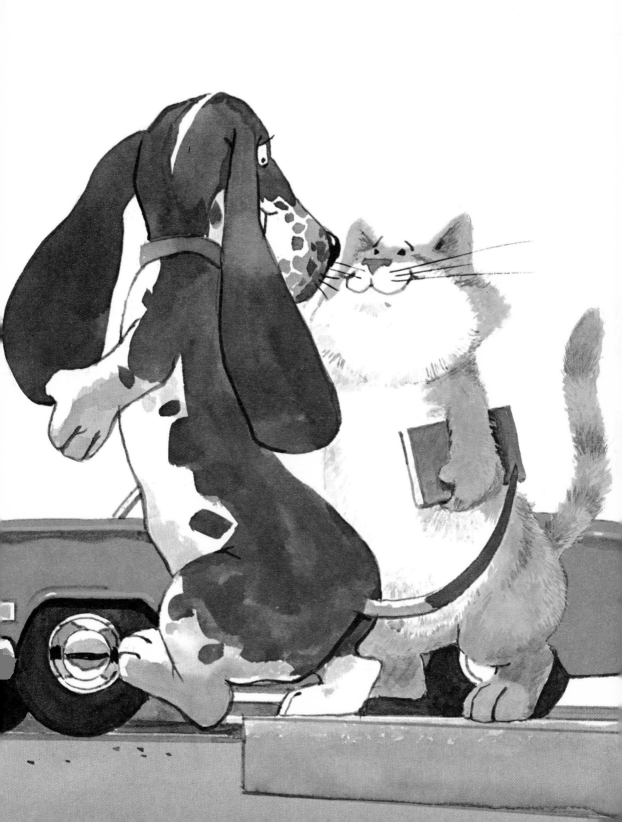

- When walking outdoors, pay attention to traffic signals.
- Stay in crosswalk.

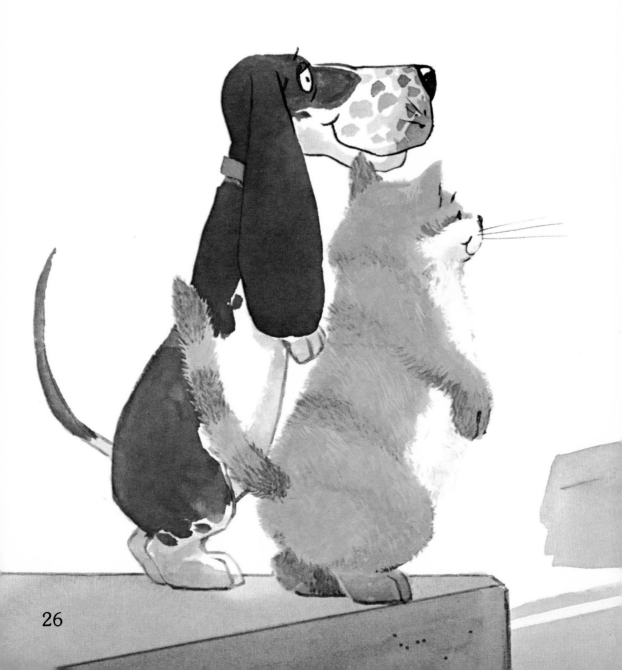

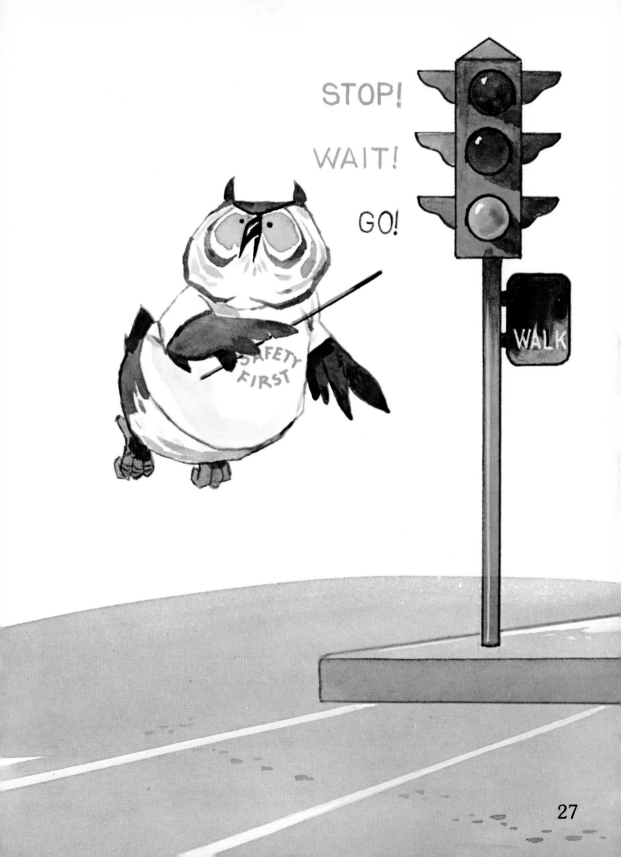

REMEMBER NOW. . . . .

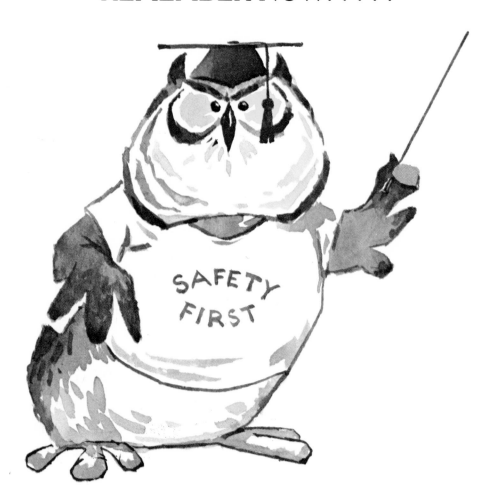

Do not play in streets.

Do not run out from between parked cars.

Cross streets only at corners.

Stop, look and listen before crossing.

Do not take dares to use play equipment in incorrect ways.

Do not play behind or near swings.

Watch for people around you when you swing a bat.

Be careful when equipment is wet and slippery.

Do not climb high fences.

Stay away from trash cans and broken bottles.

Stay away from electrical equipment.

———————————

Do not play in abandoned buildings.

Do not play or hide in old trunks or refrigerators where lid or door can swing shut, trapping you inside.

Do not stand up in a boat.

Be careful with fish hooks and knives.

Come back to shore when the water gets rough.

Look where you step when fishing on a pier.

_____

When walking outdoors, pay attention to traffic signals.

Stay in crosswalk.

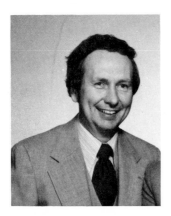

EUGENE BAKER is Vice-President for Curriculum and Materials Development, Zachary's Workshop Ltd., Lake Forest, Illinois. Dr. Baker graduated from Carthage College, Carthage, Illinois. He received his M.A. and Ph.D. in education from Northwestern University. He has worked as a teacher, as a principal, and as director of curriculum and instruction.

Gene is the author of many children's books, educational audio-visual materials, and numerous articles on reading, guidance, and learning research. One of his best-known series is the *I Want to Be* books. In addition to writing and speaking widely, he has served as consultant on various educational programs at both national and local levels. Dr. Baker also teaches Adult Sunday Church School.

Dr. Baker's practical help to schools where new programs are evolving is sparked by his boundless enthusiasm. He likes to see reading, social studies, and language arts taught with countless resources, including many books, to encourage students to think independently, creatively, and critically. Gene and his wife, Donna, live in Arlington Heights, Illinois. They have a son and two daughters.